Keto Lunch Dinners

Ketogenic Diet Lunch and Dinner Recipes

Your Free Gifts

As a way of thanking you for the purchase, I'd like to offer you 2 complimentary gifts:

- **How To Get Through Any Weight Loss Plateau While On The Ketogenic Diet:** The title is self-explanatory; if you are struggling with getting off a weight loss plateau while on the Keto diet, you will find this free gift very eye opening on what has been ailing you. Grab your copy now by clicking/tapping here or simply enter http://bit.ly/2fantonpubketo into your browser.

- **5 Pillar Life Transformation Checklist:** This short book is about life transformation, presented in bit size pieces for easy implementation. I believe that without such a checklist, you are likely to have a hard time implementing anything in this book and any other thing you set out to do religiously and sticking to it for the long haul. It doesn't matter whether your goals relate to weight loss, relationships, personal finance, investing, personal development, improving communication in your family, your overall health, finances, improving your sex life, resolving issues in your relationship, fighting PMS successfully, investing, running a successful business, traveling etc. With a checklist like this one, you can bet that anything you do will seem a lot easier to implement until the end. Therefore, even if you don't continue reading this book, at least read the one thing that will help you in every other aspect of your life. Grab your copy now by clicking/tapping here or simply enter

Ketogenic Diet Lunch and Dinner Recipes

http://bit.ly/2fantonfreebie into your browser. Your life will never be the same again (if you implement what's in this book), I promise.

PS: I'd like your feedback. If you are happy with this book, please leave a review on Amazon.

Introduction

The Ketogenic diet is without doubt the most effective weight loss diet, as it transforms the body into a fat burning machine without starving it of essential nutrients. All you do is to limit intake of carbohydrates significantly (as these make you fat), increase your intake of fats and keep your intake of proteins at a moderate level.

If you've committed to following the diet, you may have to come to terms with the fact that preparing lunches and dinners can be a bit of a hassle when you don't have a reference point for what to prepare. Sure, you may have your go-to recipes at the beginning but if you are following the diet for weeks, months or even years, you may soon run out of ideas.

That's where a cookbook comes in handy. With a cookbook specially designed for lunches and dinners, you can bet that you won't waste a lot of your valuable time trying to convert breakfast, snack and other recipes into lunches. This book goes far beyond the recipes though, as you will also learn such things like what the diet is about, its benefits, foods you are allowed to eat (you will realize it is not just salads and meats) and much more.

Let's begin.

Table of Contents

Your Free Gifts -------------------------------------- **2**

Introduction -- **4**

A Comprehensive Background To The Ketogenic Diet--------------------------------------**12**

The Role of Fat and Carbs in Weight Gain and Weight Loss--*13*

The Benefits of the Ketogenic Diet------------**18**

Ketogenic Diet Lunch and Dinner Recipes 24

Meats And Chicken-Based Lunch Recipes- 24

Keto Pizza- Grilled Chicken and Spinach --------*24*

Peanut Sauce on Beef Satay -----------------------*27*

Oven Roasted Or Grilled Cabbage Steaks With Bacon, Garlic & Lemon ----------------------------*33*

Low Carb Portabella Sliders - Keto, Gluten-Free --*36*

Cabbage Soup Recipe -----------------------------*38*

Meat Pie-- *40*

Vegetarian-Friendly Keto Recipes ----------- **43**

Roasted Garlic Cauliflower-----------------------*43*

Creamy Mash Cauliflower------------------------*45*

Coconut Lime Noodles with Chili Tamari Tofu -*47*

1: With Dairy — 50
- Low Carb Chicken Divan Casserole — 50
- Bacon Cheeseburger Casserole — 53
- Pizza Casserole — 55
- Creamy Shredded Zucchini Casserole — 57

2: Without Dairy — 59

Tuna Zoodle Casserole — 59

Creative Egg-Based Lunch Dishes — 62
- Low Carb Keto Everything Bagels — 62
- Starbucks Inspired Microwave Egg Bites — 65
- Keto Egg Fast Snickerdoodle Crepes — 68
- Salted Caramel Custard (Low Carb) — 70

Delicious And Quick Lunch Soups — 72
- Tomato Soup With Cheese Croutons — 72
- Keto No-Noodle Chicken Soup — 74
- Creamy Garlic Chicken Soup — 76
- Slow Cooker Low Carb Zuppa Toscana Soup — 78
- Keto Broccoli Cheddar Soup — 80

Breads, Pizzas And Other Meat-Free Baked Goods — 82

Keto Bread — 82
- Low-Carb Pizza — 84

Microwave Keto Bread - 90 Sec Flaxseed Bread 87

Vegetarian Keto Pizza Recipe -------------------- 90

Fish, Salads And Fish Salads ----------------- 92

Avocado BLT Salad With Sweet Onion Bacon Ranch Dressing ------------------------------------92

Five Minute Marinated Feta & Sun-Dried Tomato Salad --95

Chicken Salad Stuffed Avocado ------------------ 97

Grilled Halloumi Salad ---------------------------99

Keto Lemon Garlic Ghee Salmon With Leek Asparagus Ginger Saute ---------------------------101

Keto Baked Fish With Lemon Butter Sauce ---- 103

Best Keto Tuna Salad ------------------------------ 105

Paleo Sardine Stuffed Avocado ---------------- 107

Keto Creamy Crab Salad ---------------------- 109

Easy keto egg salad ------------------------------ 111

5 Ingredient Keto Chicken Salad ----------------113

Conclusion ---------------------------------------115

Do You Like My Book & Approach To Publishing? --116

1: First, I'd Love It If You Leave a Review of This Book on Amazon. --------------------------------116

2: Check Out My Other Keto Diet Books --------116

3: Let's Get In Touch ----------------------------118

4: Grab Some Freebies On Your Way Out; Giving Is Receiving, Right? -------------------------------- *118*

5: Suggest Topics That You'd Love Me To Cover To Increase Your Knowledge Bank. ------------ *119*

PSS: Let Me Also Help You Save Some Money! ---**120**

Copyright 2018 by Fantonpublishers.com - All rights reserved.

PS:

I have special interest in the Ketogenic diet. My wife has been following the Ketogenic diet and I can honestly say that the journey has been amazing. The diet works. And this is why I have committed to writing and publishing as many of the Ketogenic diet books as possible to give readers different options as far as the Ketogenic diet is concerned.

For instance, I have Ketogenic diet books exclusively dedicated for:

- Breakfast
- Main Meals
- Snacks
- Desserts
- Appetizers
- Soups
- Vegetarians
- Crockpot/slow cooker users
- Instant pot users
- Air fryer users
- People who are on the Paleo diet
- People who are following intermittent fasting

- People who are following carb cycling

And much more.

You can check out my [Ketogenic Diet Books fan page shop](#) for more of the books, as I continue publishing more and more. If you want me to add your category of the Ketogenic diet books that I have published so far, make sure to send me a message. I will do the heavy lifting for you and get back to you with a book that you will love.

You could also subscribe to my newsletter to receive updates whenever I have something new: http://bit.ly/2Cketodietfanton.

Amidst all the muddle in the dieting world where diets are rising and falling, the Ketogenic diet has stood the test of time. Actually, the popularity of this diet keeps rising over time and you'll see everyone –from celebrities, politicians to doctors and nutritionists -praising and endorsing it on multiple platforms. Even with all the hype that this diet has been having lately, I still wouldn't recommend adopting this diet, or any other based on all the positive reviews and popularity, as *all that could be reflective of successful advertising and marketing by its proponents.*

To support it objectively for what it is, it is important to understand why it's touted as the best diet, and that means understanding how it's structured, the science behind it and its underlying principles. This is where we will begin before getting to the recipes.

A Comprehensive Background To The Ketogenic Diet

What exactly is a Ketogenic diet?

The Ketogenic (or keto) diet is simply a diet that is composed of fats, carbohydrates and protein in different proportions than what the typical American diet, which follows the recommendations by USDA i.e. high carb, moderate protein and minimal fat intake. Instead, the diet recommends low carb intake paired with moderate protein intake and intake of high amounts of fats. More precisely, according to the diet, you should not consume more than 50 grams of carbohydrates- this should be about 5-10% of all the calories you eat. As for proteins, you should keep your intake to the 0.7-100g for every pound of body weight range - about 20% of all the calories you take. Fats should account for up to 70-75% of all the calories you eat (taking into consideration that 1g of fat produces 9 calories.

As you can see, the aim of this diet is to reduce the amount of carbohydrates in your diet as much as possible, and replace that with fat, and a moderate amount of protein.

When you look at an ordinary lunch or dinner meal closely, you'll realize that the carbohydrates take the largest share and fat usually has the least cut. For a long time, people have always been led to believe that fat makes people fat, which explains why we have always made efforts to reduce fat from our diets as much as possible.

However, science has proven that carbohydrates are actually the biggest reason people get fat, and fat helps in weight loss.

Let me explain.

The Role of Fat and Carbs in Weight Gain and Weight Loss

When you eat, the body spends the next few hours digesting everything you've eaten, absorbing it into the bloodstream, transporting the absorbed molecules and absorbing these molecules into the cells for energy production and nourishment. The type of energy that the body will run on will primarily depend on the major macronutrient taken. Nonetheless, one thing is very important; each of the 3 macronutrients is broken down at different speeds with carbohydrates being the fastest to break down followed by fats and then proteins. Given that much of the American diet is comprised of carbohydrates, it goes without saying that much of the time, the body will run on carbohydrates primarily since they are easy to break down as well in addition to being provided to the body in large quantities. What you may not know is that these carbohydrates are secretly making you to gain weight. I will explain:

When the body digests carbohydrates, it breaks them down into easy to absorb molecules known as sugar or glucose. This glucose is then absorbed into the bloodstream for transportation to different parts of the body where the cells need it. When glucose is absorbed into the bloodstream, the presence of glucose signals the beta cells of the pancreas to secrete insulin, a hormone, whose job is to help the cells to take up glucose by triggering the insulin receptors on different cells. When the insulin receptors detect the presence of insulin in the bloodstream, they signal the cells to sort of open its doors so as to take up the available glucose. Insulin will keep the doors to the cells open to take up glucose as long as there is glucose available in the bloodstream. However, as you are well aware, the cells don't need an unlimited amount of energy; they have their limits and when that limit is reached, insulin signals the liver to start converting any extra glucose into glycogen. This glycogen is then stored in the liver and muscle cells. The body will store up to 2000 kcal of energy in form of glucose. If this limit is reached, the liver converts the excess into fatty acids and glycerol, which are then transported to different fat stores around the body to be stored as triglycerides. As you can guess, this process can make you fat if it takes place over a long time. In fact, you are considered to be in a state of constant storing of fat if your diet primarily consists of carbohydrates because insulin favors energy storage and inhibits the metabolism of fat. The only way to get your body to burn fat is to reverse the process of storing fat i.e. make sure the body is not in a fat storing mode and this is best done through either fasting or through starving your body of carbohydrates. This is where the Ketogenic diet comes in.

When you restrict your intake of carbohydrates by adopting a ketogenic diet, your body perceives this as lack of enough food. It first uses up much of the available dietary glucose, something which in turn results to a significant reduction in insulin levels. With reduced insulin levels, the body's 'starvation' hormones kick in. These hormones will prompt the body to start using stored glycogen and fats, starting with glycogen. Glycogen stores are usually the first ones to get converted back to glucose with the help of the hormone glucagon, which is secreted by the alpha cells of the pancreas, followed by the fat once the glycogen stores start reducing to significantly low levels. This process also takes place with the help of glucagon along with other hormones such as the human growth hormone. The body doesn't use up all the glycogen though; it will hold on to some before they can be all used up; these will be used to supply the body with small amounts of glucose for those glucose dependent processes like in some parts of the brain. This means the process of metabolizing stored body fat starts even before the body can deplete its glycogen stores.

What happens is that with reduced insulin levels, the 'grip' that insulin had on fats is reduced, which essentially means they are free to move around. For starters, they are transported to the liver for breakdown where they will be used for energy.

When fats get to the liver, they are broken down into fatty acids and glycerol.

Many body cells can use fatty acids for energy production. However, the brain cannot use such especially because fatty acids are not water soluble, which means they cannot cross the blood brain barrier. Glucose is water soluble, which explains why the brain prefers to use glucose. But since glucose levels are very limited on a Ketogenic diet, the body has to find an alternative. It does that by breaking down the fatty acids further in a series of processes that end up producing energy molecules referred to as ketone bodies.

More specifically, a process known as gluconeogenesis takes place where the glycerol is converted into glucose. Another process known as ketogenesis also takes place where the fatty acids are broken down into ketone bodies known acetoacetate. Acetoacetate is then further broken down into two other types of ketone bodies namely:

- Beta-hydroxybutyrate (BHB).

- Acetone

After a few weeks when you've become keto-adapted, your body will start converting acetoacetate into BHB since it is a much more efficient source of fuel than acetoacetate (it goes through an extra chemical reaction that facilitates the production of this energy for the cells). Experts will tell you that your body and brain prefer using BHB and its precursor, acetoacetate for energy simply because the cells can be able to use it more efficiently than glucose by about 70 percent.

Well, for the acetone, the body can either excrete it as waste or metabolize some of it into glucose.

In the end, and as you would expect, you gain lots of energy, which leads to improved performance, your brain function improves (as your brain receives more sustainable, efficient energy from ketones) and you lose weight!

You are said to be at optimal nutritional ketosis when the body's blood ketone levels range between **1.0mmol/L and 3.0mmol/L.** You can use a blood ketone meter to determine this.

With this diet, you can expect to experience a number of benefits when you get into ketosis.

The Benefits of the Ketogenic Diet

By now, you know how the Ketogenic diet works if you didn't understand it, and I believe you are set to start cooking for a healthier life. You might however be wondering what good these meals REALLY are to your life, and whether they are worth all the effort (especially if cooking is not your hobby). If you are new to Ketogenic dieting, let me assure you that you have made the right choice choosing this path, which is full of long-term benefits which have been venerated by people practicing it, and upheld by science. Let me state a few:

1. *You lose weight*

You already know how the diet does it. It turns you into a fat burning machine that uses fat as fuel instead of carbs as fuel. As you lose more weight, you gain confidence, flexibility and many other things -but above all, a vital sense of self-fulfillment.

2. *You stay young for long, and feel young for longer*

Ever heard of oxidative stress? If you have, you most probably know that it is not a good thing at all. Oxidative stress refers to the imbalance that exists between the production of different free radicals and the body's ability to offset or detoxify their damaging effects through neutralization with the aid of antioxidants. Free radicals are molecules containing oxygen that react highly with other molecules because they (free radicals) have unpaired electrons.

Oxidative stress makes you age quickly. Keeping the oxidative stress levels low is a great way to keep you young, and a keto diet helps with that. For one, the diet reduces the insulin levels and makes sure there is a constant supply of ketones throughout the body, which are used by the body as fuel. Reduction in insulin levels has been associated with reduced oxidative stress levels. As we discussed at the beginning of this book, a keto diet reduces insulin levels in the blood by reducing carbs in the diet, and also facilitates the creation of ketones which your body then uses as fuel.

A Ketogenic also boosts your body's production of a strong antioxidant known as uric acid, which as you may already guess, can help with reducing oxidative stress. We have countless reports today that are suggesting that the ketone bodies that this diet produces do provide a relief for, and reverses quite a number of neurological disorders that are caused by oxidative stress such as ALS, Parkinson's disease and Alzheimer's disease. This page and this one too contains all the information you need in that regard.

There is famous study that has already associated the ketone body known as Betahydroxybutyrate to decelerated aging. Apparently, it does so by triggering a gene expression that alters the factors linked with aging.

Lastly, Ketogenic diet has been said to a boost in the levels of mitochondrial glutathione, an antioxidant in the body that improves the function of the powerhouses in your cells known as mitochondria. The mitochondria create energy for your body. When this function is improved, your body can only become more revitalized and this is where you start feeling more energetic and vital.

3. Helps with diabetes

When you have diabetes, it means that your blood has high levels of blood sugar, and despite the efforts by your body to produce insulin to reduce the blood sugar, the blood sugar still remains extremely high. The problem usually starts when you continue stuffing an already glucose-rich blood with more carbs hence forcing your body to produce more and more insulin to take care of the constantly excess glucose in your blood. Sometimes, this leads to a condition known as insulin resistance where your body no longer responds to insulin, as it should and as a result, you need more insulin than you would otherwise do to control your blood sugar.

Following a Ketogenic diet helps a lot here because it gradually reduces the amount of glucose in your blood (since you are now generally taking less carbs and avoiding unhealthy carbs). As your blood sugar levels go down, your insulin reduces as well. What makes this process sustainable is the fact that you are no longer dependent on the carbs so you will not have any reason to take them anyway. With less carbs, your weight also reduces which is also good news here because weight gain is also a risk factor for diabetes.

4. Reduces the risk of heart disease and helps maintain a strong cardiovascular health.

Contrary to what most of us have heard, high fat diets (such as the Ketogenic diet) don't increase the amount of cholesterol in the body and clog the arteries; they actually optimize your cholesterol levels and improve your heart health.

To understand how this happens, consider a type of lipid or fat found in the body known as triglycerides. These fatty acids store energy for later use. They can be broken down into different fatty acids as well as glycerol to fuel the body, with the latter being broken further into glucose for energy. With increased triglycerides in your blood, you are at risk of developing cardiovascular illnesses, diabetes and other chronic diseases. When you consistently consume carbs (especially processed or refined carbs), the body produces insulin in response to the glucose released into the bloodstream, and the insulin converts the glucose into triglycerides. The Ketogenic diet helps manage this by ensuring you cut on the carbs.

Secondly, consider a class of lipids known as cholesterol. These compounds build hormones such as the testosterone and maintain the integrity of cell membranes among many other functions. Under cholesterol, we have High density lipoprotein (HDL) or the 'good cholesterol'. HDL specifically collects unusable cholesterol around the body and takes it to the liver to be destroyed or recycled so that it doesn't accumulate and clog the arteries. HDL also has anti-inflammatory effects, and has been conjectured to be the one responsible for reducing inflammatory activity by regulating microphages (immune system cells). Scientists have thus spent years looking for a way of increasing HDL cholesterol in the body, and Ketogenic diet has been considered one of the best solutions yet. There was a meta-analysis that was recently published in the British Journal of Nutrition. The research looked at the impact of the Ketogenic diet on key cardiovascular health metrics, which includes HDL cholesterol. All the 13 randomized controlled studies had as many as 1,415 subjects and took place for a full year. The subjects who were assigned a Ketogenic diet had an increase of HDL (0.12 mmol/L), which was asserted to be twice the average HDL increase of the low-fat dieters which was at 0.06 mmol/L.

It thus goes without saying that a ketogenic diet could be your best bet when it comes to improving your cardiovascular health as it improves the levels of HDL in your body.

Other benefits include:

- Better management of cancer
- Better mood
- Reduced depression and anxiety
- Better brain function
- Improved immunity
- Reduced appetite
- Enhanced performance in sports
- And a lot more that you will only discover by following the Ketogenic diet and measuring your progress using

the Ketone meter to ensure you actually get into optimal ketosis and stay in it.

Bottom line: The list is endless, as you probably already know. If you are new (or haven't ever tried it), get started today to understand what I'm talking about ☺

In the next part of the book, we will focus on the different recipes you can prepare for lunch and dinner to ensure you don't have to rely on the same old recipes over and over again.

Ketogenic Diet Lunch and Dinner Recipes

PS: For easy reading and navigation, I have categorized the recipes for you based on the nature of the recipe, the main ingredients and such.

Let's start with eats and chicken based recipes.

Meats And Chicken-Based Lunch Recipes

Keto Pizza- Grilled Chicken and Spinach

Serves 2

Ingredients

1 boneless, skinless, chicken breast

1 clove garlic, minced

1/4 teaspoon xanthan gum thickener

1/2 cup part skim, shredded mozzarella

1/2 tablespoon olive oil

1/2 cup half & half (which I used) or heavy whipping cream. Nutrition facts may change if you use anything else

1 cup fresh spinach, roughly chopped

Sea salt & pepper to taste

For the fathead dough, use:

2 oz. cream cheese

1 egg, beaten

1/3 cup almond flour

3/4 cup shredded mozzarella

1/4 teaspoon garlic powder

Directions

Do the following to make the pizza crust:

Melt the cream cheese and mozzarella in your oven for 30 seconds at a time while mixing often. Mix the beaten egg with almond flour and the rest of the dough ingredients in another bowl. Mix the flour with the cheese mixture well until you reach a sticky dough consistency.

Refrigerate as you prepare the chicken and sauce.

Sauté the chicken over medium heat in a skillet until it is ready. Remove it and set aside. Next, boil the garlic along with the xantham gum with half and half in the skillet and when you notice the chicken starting to thicken, reduce to simmer.

Fold it in the spinach and cook until it wilts. Work out the dough on your pizza pan using your hands and bake for 10 more minutes at 350 degrees F. You must ensure the crust is pre-baked to be able to hold up to the toppings and the sauce. Now spread the mixture of spinach and sauce nicely onto your cooked pizza crust and top using the shredded cheese and chicken.

Bake until the cheese melts, which is about 5 minutes. If your microwave oven and crust weren't already hot from making the dough, you can instead bake for 10 minutes.

Leave it to cool for a couple of minutes before cutting it into four pieces.

Nutritional information per serving

Calories: 687

Fat: 54.2 g

Carbs: 11.2 g

Protein: 43.2 g

Peanut Sauce on Beef Satay

Serves 4

Ingredients

For the beef Satay and Marinade

1 pound flank steak or skirt steak

2 tablespoons tamari Soy Sauce or coconut aminos

1/2 teaspoon ground coriander

2 tablespoons Red Boat Fish Sauce or your favorite

2 tablespoons Sukrin Gold powdered (coconut sugar, swerve Confection or honey)

For the Thai Peanut Sauce

1/4 cup smooth almond butter or peanut butter

1/3 cup of coconut milk full fat from a can

1-2 teaspoons Chile garlic sauce

1/2 teaspoon Thai Red Curry Paste e.g. Mae Ploy

1 tablespoon Sukrin Gold, powdered (you can as well use honey or coconut sugar)

Additions

1 tablespoon olive oil to apply on the meat before grilling

Foil to prevent the skewers from burning

In bamboo skewers. These should be soaked for a few hours in water

Directions

If you're using the Sukrin Gold, powder all the 3 tablespoons.

Cut the flank steak into strips measuring 1 ½ inches such that the meat grain goes across the strip horizontally. Stick the skewers into the meat to leave a handle that is long enough to hold during eating. Combine the soy sauce, fish sauce and the sweetener together in a baking dish and ensure you coat all the beef surfaces. Sprinkle the meat using the coriander, rub it in and leave to marinate for 15 to 20 minutes. In the meantime, shake the coconut milk can, preheat your grill and embark on the peanut sauce.

Get a small-medium microwavable bowl, add in the peanut butter and place it in the microwave for a couple of seconds. Stir the Chile garlic sauce, the Thai red curry paste and sweetener of your choice using a small whisk. Add the coconut milk to the mixture bit by bit, stirring in between with the whisk.

NOTE: if you are planning on making a cucumber salad, the time to do so is now.

Next, pour one tablespoon of oil on the beef, making sure to coat all surfaces. Fold a piece of foil in half to place beneath the skewers' handles as you cook on the grill. Remove the beef from the marinade and put it on the grill to cook. Line them up and put the foil beneath the handles. Grill on both sides until it's done. This will however depend on the thickness of your meat and how hot your grill can get.

Serve the beef satay either with regular salad, Thai Chicken Coconut Soup or Thai cucumber with an Asian dressing of your choice.

Nutritional information per serving

Calories: 373

Fat: 27 g

Carbs: 4 g

Protein: 28 g

Creamy Cauliflower Mac and Cheese with Ham

Serves 4

Ingredients

1 pound cauliflower

3 slices reduced sodium bacon

1 teaspoon garlic

1/4 cup dry white wine

2 oz. cream cheese

1 cup cheddar cheese (4 oz.)

1/4 teaspoon white pepper

10 oz. ham, cubed

1/4 cup (1 oz.) onion

1 teaspoon organic chicken base

1/4 cup water

1/2 cup mozzarella cheese (2 oz.)

1 teaspoon Worcestershire sauce

Directions

Cut the cauliflower into tiny florets and steam them until they are tender. Drain well and leave them uncovered for the steam to escape.

Meanwhile, chop the onions and bacon, mince the garlic and cube the ham.

Add your bacon to a medium-large pan and cook over medium heat until crispy. Remove the bacon and pour the fat out but leave enough to coat the pan.

Sauté the garlic and onions for 2 minutes, or until softened. Add water, some wine, cream cheese and chicken base, making sure to stir occasionally to have the cheese properly melted.

After that, add the mozzarella, cheddar, white pepper and Worcestershire sauce, and gently simmer until the cheese melts and the sauce becomes thick and nice.

Add the ham and drained cauliflower to the pan and heat through for a short while and top with bacon. Serve.

You can alternatively spoon it into a serving dish and then top with the bacon.

Note that the sauce becomes thickest when it is left to cool a bit before serving. The left-overs should be refrigerated.

Reheating

When you want to reheat, put the cheese casserole and leftover mac in a microwavable bowl, cover and cook- stirring halfway through. The cooking times may vary depending on how much cauliflower casserole is left over, as well as your microwave's power.

Alternatively, you can cover the casserole with foil and cook it in a moderately hot oven (this is about 350 degrees F) until hot. Just ensure you stir at least once. Again, the cooking times may vary depending on the manner in which you are reheating the cauliflower casserole, and the size of your oven.

Nutritional information per serving

Calories: 404

Fat: 28 g

Carbs: 8.7 g

Protein: 27 g

Oven Roasted Or Grilled Cabbage Steaks With Bacon, Garlic & Lemon

Serves 8

Ingredients

8 slices bacon

8 cloves minced garlic

2 tablespoons lemon juice

1/2 teaspoon sea salt

1 head cabbage

1/4 cup olive oil

1/2 teaspoon black pepper

Directions

For the cabbage steak marinade:

Put the bacon slices on a large pan. Set your stove to medium low heat and place the pan on it. Fry the bacon until crispy, for roughly 8-10 minutes, and flip as needed.

Meanwhile, cut the cabbage into slices that are 2 cm thick.

Add the lemon juice, olive oil, black pepper and sea salt to a sizeable re-sealable plastic bag and mix well.

Remove the bacon and set it aside so that it drains, so that the bacon fat is left in the pan. Now add the minced garlic and sauté for a minute or so, until it is fragrant.

Give the pan containing the bacon fat some 5 to 10 minutes to cool so that it does not melt the plastic bag. When the bacon fat cools enough, pour the fat into the bag. Scoop the garlic that is left over using a spatula and add it to the mix; seal and mix properly to create the marinade.

Now put the cabbage steaks into the marinade bag and coat well. Refrigerate for not less than half an hour.

For the grilled cabbage steaks:

Preheat your grill at medium heat

Take between 4 and 8 minutes to grill the cabbage streaks on both sides, until they are crispy and tender around the edges.

Top with cooked bacon to serve and garnish with parsley if you want.

For oven roasted cabbage steaks:

Preheat your oven to 425 degrees F.

Get a large baking sheet and grease it properly. Remember that you can line it with parchment paper or foil if you desire. Place the cabbage steaks nicely in one layer.

Roast the cabbage steaks in the oven for 30-35 minutes until crispy and tender around the edges.

Top with some cooked bacon and if you want, garnish with parsley.

Serve and enjoy!

Nutritional information per serving

Calories: 184

Fat: 15 g

Carbs: 6 g

Protein: 4g

Low Carb Portabella Sliders - Keto, Gluten-Free

Yields 12 sliders

Ingredients

1 pound grass fed beef (80/20 is ideal for burgers)

2 dill pickles, sliced

12 basil leaves

4 slices of sharp cheddar that have been sliced into quarters

Salt and pepper to taste

24 baby portabella mushrooms

4 tablespoons chopped yellow onion

2 tablespoons extra-virgin olive oil

Yellow mustard, mayo, sriracha or low carb ketchup (optional)

Directions

Remove all the stems from the portabella mushroom caps and the wipe with a damp paper towel properly to get rid of any debris or dirt. Heat a tablespoon of olive oil in a tiny saucepan, over medium heat. Add the mushroom caps and cook for 2 minutes on each of the sides to allow the mushrooms to cook through, but also retain their firmness.

Remove the mushrooms from the pan and place them on paper towels to let the liquid drain off. Divide the ground pepper into 12 parts, and roll each one of them in a tiny disc shape. Add pepper and salt to taste. Heat the remaining tablespoon of olive oil over medium heat. When the pan becomes sufficiently hot, add the meat and let it cook for three minutes on one side. Flip to cook on the other side for three more minutes. You can cook to the level of doneness you desire.

Now stack a mushroom, then burger and cheese, onion and pickles, and finally your favorite condiments. You can top with another mushroom cap and then garnish a leaf of basil. Use a toothpick to hold it in place.

Serve.

Nutritional information per serving (one slider)

Calories: 267

Fat: 20.1 g

Carbs: 1.3 g

Protein: 10.4 g

Cabbage Soup Recipe

Serves 10

Ingredients

2 pounds ground beef- 90% lean

1 clove garlic minced

1 head cabbage large, chopped

10 oz. diced tomatoes & green chilies (1 can)

Salt and pepper to taste

1/4 onion large, diced

1 teaspoon cumin ground

4 cubes bouillon

4 cups water

Directions

Brown the beef over medium heat and then add the onion. Let it cook until it turns translucent.

Put the beef and onion into a stock pot and then add the cabbage, diced tomatoes and green chilies, garlic, bouillon cubes, cumin and water to the pot.

Combine the ingredients properly and leave it to boil over high heat.

Reduce the heat to medium-low and cover. Let it simmer for 30 to 45 minutes.

Serve and enjoy!

Nutritional information per serving

Calories: 261

Fat: 18 g

Carbs: 6 g

Protein: 17 g

Meat Pie

Serves 6

Ingredients

½ yellow onion, finely chopped

2 tablespoons of olive oil or butter

Salt and pepper

4 tablespoons tomato paste/ ajvar relish

1 garlic clove, finely chopped

20 oz. ground beef or ground lamb

1 tablespoon dried basil or dried oregano

½ cup water

For the pie crust

¾ cup almond flour

4 tablespoons sesame seeds

4 tablespoons coconut flour

1 tablespoon ground psyllium husk powder

1 teaspoon baking powder

1 pinch salt

3 tablespoons olive oil or coconut oil

1 egg

4 tablespoons water

For the topping:

7 oz. shredded cheese

8 oz. cottage cheese

Directions

Preheat your oven to 350 degrees F.

Heat butter or olive oil and fry the garlic and onion for a few minutes, over medium heat, until the onion becomes soft. Now add the ground beef and continue frying. Now add basil or oregano, and then pepper and salt to taste.

Add pesto, tomato paste and then water. Reduce the heat and leave it to simmer for at least 20 minutes. Make dough for the crust while the meat simmers.

Add all the dough ingredients to a powerful food processor and mix until the dough forms a ball. You can also mix the dough ingredients by hand using a fork if you don't have a food processor.

Now grease a 9- 10 inch wide spring form pan and then line it with a piece of parchment paper. This will make it easier to remove the pie when it gets done. Note that you can also use a deep-dish pie pan to achieve the same. Spread the dough evenly in the pan and nicely up along the sides using well-greased fingers or a spatula.

Bake the crust for between 10 and 15 minutes, take it out and put the meat in the crust. Mix the shredded cheese and cottage cheese together and place it on top of the pie.

Bake for between 30 and 40 minutes on the lower rack, or until you notice the color of the pie changed to a golden color.

Serve with some fresh green salad and dressing.

Nutritional information per serving

Calories: 622

Fat: 47g

Carbs: 7g

Protein: 38g

Vegetarian-Friendly Keto Recipes

Roasted Garlic Cauliflower

Serves 4

Ingredients

1 medium head cauliflower

1/2 teaspoon sea salt

4 cloves garlic or more, minced

1/4 cup avocado oil (you can also use light olive oil)

1/4 teaspoon black pepper

Directions

First of all, preheat your oven to 400 degrees F. Apply grease on a non-stick baking sheet, or line it with a foil and then grease it.

Slice the cauliflower into slices measuring 1.25 centimeters in thickness, and then cut them into tinier florets.

Add the cauliflower to a large bowl and toss it with sea salt, oil, minced garlic and black pepper.

Place the cauliflower on the baking sheet in a single layer.

Bake for between 15 and 20 minutes until the bottom area turns golden. Flip it and bake it for between 5-10 more minutes until it turns golden on the bottom area again.

Nutritional information per serving

Calories: 161

Fat: 14g

Carbs: 5g

Protein: 2g

Creamy Mash Cauliflower

Serves 4

Ingredients

5 cups cauliflower, chopped

3 tablespoons butter

2 teaspoon dried rosemary

1/2 teaspoon pepper

4 tablespoons heavy whipping cream

5 cloves garlic, minced

3 tablespoons parmesan

Pink Salt

Directions

Chop five cups of cauliflower.

Boil a pot of water- the water should be enough to cover the entire cauliflower. Now add the cauliflower and boil for about 15 minutes, or until they become tender.

Drain the cauliflower well and add to a processor.

Get a saucepan, add the rosemary and garlic and cook over medium heat until fragrant.

Add the garlic, melted butter and rosemary to your processor and pulse a few times until it becomes properly combined.

Add the parmesan, cream, pepper and salt to the processor. Process until creamy and smooth. Before serving, you might want to taste for the salt level.

Serve warm.

Nutritional information per serving

Calories: 173.75

Fat: 15.25g

Carbs: 3.75g

Protein: 4g

Coconut Lime Noodles with Chili Tamari Tofu

Serves 4

Ingredients

<u>Noodles</u>

1 can full-fat coconut milk (13.5oz)

1/2 teaspoon ground or fresh grated ginger

2 packages shirataki noodles (8oz)

1/4 teaspoon red pepper flakes

4 tablespoons sesame seeds

Pinch of salt

Juice and zest of 1 lime

<u>Tofu</u>

1 block extra firm tofu (13.5oz)

1 tablespoon olive oil

4 tablespoons low sodium tamari

1/4 teaspoon cayenne pepper (or any desired ground chili pepper)

Directions

Pre-heat the oven to 350 degrees F.

Drain the tofu, and press out the excess moisture, and cube it into blocks measuring 1"x1".

Combine together the cayenne, olive oil and tamari. Arrange the tofu cubes in one layer in a shallow dish and then pour the mixture over the tofu. You will also want to flip the pieces a couple of times so that they are covered evenly.

Put the pieces of tofu on a baking sheet and then bake for 20-25 minutes.

As the tofu bakes, rinse and drain the noodles. Add to a pan on medium heat, together with the rest of the noodle ingredients and then mix properly until well integrated. Cover partially and cook for 10 more minutes and then reduce the heat and keep cooking for yet another 10 minutes.

When the tofu is set, turn off the heat and leave everything to cool for a couple of minutes.

Garnish the dish with red pepper flakes, lime zest, microgreens, sesame seeds or anything else your heart may desire.

Nutritional information per serving:

Calories: 374

Fat: 31.1g

Carbs: 9.1g

Protein: 15.7g

Delightful Casseroles

1: With Dairy

Low Carb Chicken Divan Casserole

Serves 6

Ingredients

3 tablespoons ghee or butter

1/2 tablespoon minced garlic

1 cup chicken stock (or broth)

3 cups frozen cauliflower or riced cauliflower

1 teaspoon lemon juice

3 cups steamed, chopped broccoli

A pinch of parsley

2 boneless chicken breasts

1 small yellow onion

1/2 teaspoon garlic salt

10 cranks of cracked black pepper

1 cup heavy cream

1/2 cup mayonnaise

2 cups shredded cheddar cheese

Ketogenic Diet Lunch and Dinner Recipes

Ingredients

Preheat your oven to 350 degrees F.

Put the two chicken breasts in a pot halfway filled with water.

Cook on high and let it boil until the chicken cooks through- this should be about 180 degrees.

As that happens, cook up the onions and garlic in a frying pan with the ghee over low heat. Meanwhile, add your cauliflower to a food processor or a blender and blend it up for a few seconds until it looks like rice.

After two or so minutes after the onions have begun cooking, start adding in the spices bit by bit, as you mix them with the onions as you go.

After about two minutes of the onions cooking, begin adding in the spices one at a time, mixing them into the onions as you go.

Add the cauliflower immediately the onions become soft.

When the cauliflower itself becomes soft, add the chicken broth and cook tightly covered for roughly 10 minutes.

Check on the boiling chicken; if it's reached 180 degrees, take it out and set it aside.

Now add the lemon juice and cream, uncover and let it simmer for roughly 10 minutes on low. As it simmers, mix it a couple of times to ensure it doesn't burn below.

Next, add in the mayo, mix and then switch off the burner. Get a fork and begin pulling the chicken apart. Add half of this chicken into the mixture of cauliflower cream. Line the bottom of your casserole dish with the other half. Add the steamed, chopped broccoli on top of the chicken in a layer and on top of it, add the cauliflower cream mixture. Top with some cheddar cheese and then cover tinfoil; put it in your oven for half an hour. Remove the tinfoil and cook for another 10 minutes.

Nutritional information per serving

Calories: 317

Fat: 22g

Carbs: 6g

Protein: 22g

Bacon Cheeseburger Casserole

Serves 12

Ingredients

2 pounds of ground beef

1/2 teaspoon of powdered onion

8 eggs

1 cup heavy cream

1/4 teaspoon ground pepper

2 cloves large garlic

1 pound of cooked and chopped "no sugar" bacon

1 can tomato paste (6 oz.)

1/2 teaspoon salt

12 ounces grated cheddar cheese, divided

Instructions

Brown the ground beef with onion powder and garlic.

Drain the excess grease and then lay the beef on a casserole pan.

Stir the pieces of bacon into the cooked beef.

Next, get a medium bowl, add the eggs, heavy cream, tomato paste, pepper and salt and whisk well until they combine well.

Add 8 ounces of grated cheese into the egg mixture and then pour the egg mixture over the bacon and beef and stir.

Top with the rest of the grated cheese.

Bake for 30-35 minutes at 350 degrees F. It should be golden brown on top.

NOTE: if you want to have a casserole that contains less eggs, you can reduce the eggs and add more beef. Also, onions, pickles and mushrooms are awesome add-ins!

Nutritional information per serving

Calories: 587

Fat: 49g

Carbs: 4g

Protein: 29g

Pizza Casserole

Serves 6

Ingredients

1 little eggplant sliced into strips, about 2" wide

5 oz. shredded parmesan

4 oz. pizza sauce

8 oz. mozzarella cheese, shredded

3/4 lb. spicy Italian pork sausage crumble, cooked.

1 tablespoon coconut oil

Directions

Grease your pan using the coconut oil and then line the eggplant strips on it. You should ideally have one layer –you might have more though.

Spread the pizza sauce in a light layer over the eggplant. Top with half of the parmesan and mozzarella.

After that, add the pork sausage and add half of the remaining parmesan and mozzarella as topping.

Spread some marinara over it and place it in your oven for one hour, at 350 degrees.

Just before the pizza is done (about six minutes), take out the pan from the oven and spread the remaining parmesan over it. Garnish with the Italian parsley.

Nutritional information per serving

Calories: 431

Fat: 32g

Carbs: 7g

Protein: 27g

Creamy Shredded Zucchini Casserole

Serves 6

Ingredients

26 oz. zucchini, grated

4 ounces cream cheese cubed

Pepper to taste

2 tablespoons butter cubed

1/4 teaspoon sea salt

2 tablespoons Parmesan cheese shredded

Directions

Grate the zucchini if you have to and place in clean kitchen towel to squeeze out excess water.

Put the shredded zucchini in a baking pan measuring 8 x 8 inch/ 7 x 11 inches and then dot the butter over the zucchini evenly.

Bake it for about 15 minutes without covering- at 350 degrees F.

Add some cream cheese, pepper and salt and stir until the cheese melts. Smooth the top and sprinkle the parmesan evenly on top of it.

Bake uncovered for 5 more minutes.

NOTE: you can sprinkle the top with crushed pork rinds instead of using parmesan cheese, or together with it.

Nutritional information per serving

Calories: 118

Fat: 11g

Carbs: 3g

Protein: 3g

2: Without Dairy

Tuna Zoodle Casserole

Serves 3 – 4

Ingredients

1 large zucchini

1/2 cup diced onion

3 large mushrooms

1 teaspoon salt

1 tablespoon lemon juice

1 broccoli crown

2/3 cup cashew cream

2 cans tuna, in water

1 minced garlic clove

1 teaspoon mustard

1 teaspoon black pepper

1/2 teaspoon dried rosemary

2-3 tablespoons mayo

1/2 cup chopped pecans (or walnuts, or cashews)

Instructions

First of all, ensure you have your cashew cream and mayo ready.

Preheat your oven to 325 degrees F. Next, zoodle your zucchini and then place the zoodles flat on your kitchen towel and sprinkle with salt. Allow them to rest here as they release their liquid as you prepare the rest. Mince the onion and garlic, and add in to the casserole dish.

Slice the mushrooms thinly and add to the dish as well.

Drain the tuna cans and place the tuna in the casserole dish. Add one tablespoon of mayo, rosemary, mustard, lemon juice, salt and pepper and mix properly.

Wrap the towel around the zucchini and press the water out.

Now add the zoodles to the dish and then toss to mix.

Pour the cashew cream in as you mix gently.

Cut the broccoli crown into florets and them mince them into quarter inch pieces, and then toss with the chopped pecans in a bowl. Finally, mix with the rest of the mayo.

Spread this mix over the casserole and sprinkle with salt lightly.

Bake in the oven for about 30 minutes. The top should be toasty and the inside should be creamy. Ensure you use a knife to cut the pieces before your serve, otherwise the zoodles might pull out the entire thing!

Nutritional information per serving

Ketogenic Diet Lunch and Dinner Recipes

Calories: 272

Fat: 20.7g

Carbs: 8.1g

Protein: 14.6g

Creative Egg-Based Lunch Dishes

Low Carb Keto Everything Bagels

Makes 6 Bagels

Ingredients

2 cups almond flour

1 teaspoon onion powder

3 large eggs, divided

5 tablespoons cream cheese

1 teaspoon garlic powder

1 teaspoon dried Italian seasoning

3 cups shredded low moisture mozzarella cheese

3 tablespoons Everything Bagel Seasoning (you can get the recipe here)

Directions

Preheat your oven to 425 degrees and then line some parchment paper on a rimmed baking sheet. Sipat can also work.

Combine the baking powder, almond flour, onion powder, garlic powder and Italian seasoning and mix until well combined. You can pour the mixture through a flour sifter to make sure all the baking powder combines fully with the other ingredients.

Next, crack one egg into a little bowl and whisk using a fork. You'll use this egg as the egg wash for the bagel top. You will add the rest of the eggs to the dough.

Mix the cream cheese and mozzarella cheese in a large microwave safe mixing bowl. Microwave for one and a half minutes and then remove. Stir to combine and take it back into the oven for one more minute. Mix until it combines properly.

Add the other two eggs to the mixing bowl along with the almond flour mixture. Combine properly until you are satisfied with the incorporation of all ingredients. If you notice the dough having some stringy texture which is basically unworkable, just place it back into the microwave and leave it for 30 seconds to soften a bit and resume the mixing.

Split the dough into six equal portions, and roll each one of them into a ball.

Press your finger into the center of each one of them to form a ring of some sort. Stretch these rings to create a tiny hole in the middle of each one and create bagel shapes out of them.

Using the egg wash, brush the top of all the bagels and top them with the 'everything bagel seasoning'.

Place in the middle rack and bake until golden brown, which is about 12 - 14 minutes.

Nutritional information per serving

Calories: 449

Fat: 35.5g

Carbs: 6g

Protein: 27.8g

Starbucks Inspired Microwave Egg Bites

Serves 1

Ingredients

2 eggs

1/4 cup 2% cottage cheese (63g)

1/2 slice provolone (10g)

1/8 teaspoon salt

2 tablespoon cheddar cheese (15g)

1 teaspoon butter (5g)

1/8 teaspoon pepper

For the topping:

1/2 slice provolone

1-2 slices bacon

Directions

Find a dish or loaf pan in which 2 small cups or ramekins will fit and place them inside the dish.

Grease the ramekins using oil.

Blend all the base ingredients in a food processor until they are smooth. It's completely fine if there are tiny flecks of cheese.

Cook a slice of bacon until it turns crispy, and then drain on a paper towel and set aside.

Now pour the mixture through a sieve of a fine colander into all the greased ramekins, ensuring to distribute the mixture evenly. In case there are any cheese bits left over, you can simply scoop them all into the ramekins as well. The sieve in this case will help get rid of any air bubbles.

If you want, you can break the slice of bacon in half, and reserve the other half. Sprinkle tiny pieces of it into all the ramekins on top of the egg mixture.

Boil one cup of water and add it to the dish surrounding the ramekins. Get a saran wrap and cover the whole thing.

Microwave for 4 minutes and 30 seconds, and let it sit in the microwave for 2 minutes afterward, with the door well shut to finish setting. As microwaves can vary, add more or less time considering how much you would like your eggs cooked. After the 4 minutes and 30 seconds, my eggs were quite smooth and soft.

Now get some mitts or tongs and remove from the microwave; get the ramekins off the water bath and leave to cool for a couple of minutes before removing the egg bites from all the ramekins gently, using a knife. Turn them upside-down onto a plate.

Use a bit of cheese (such as provolone) and bacon to top each egg bite.

Nutritional information per serving

Ketogenic Diet Lunch and Dinner Recipes

Calories: 442

Fat: 34g

Carbs: 3g

Protein: 31g

Keto Egg Fast Snickerdoodle Crepes

Serves 4

Ingredients

6 eggs

1 teaspoon cinnamon

Butter for frying

5 oz. cream cheese, softened

1 tablespoon granulated sugar substitute (such as swerve, splenda and ideal)

Use the following for the filling:

8 tablespoon butter, softened

1 tablespoon (or more) cinnamon

1/3 cup granulated sugar substitute

Directions

Add all the first five ingredients apart from the butter to a blender and blend until smooth. Leave the batter to settle for five minutes.

Add the butter to a nonstick pan and heat it over medium heat until it starts sizzling.

Add batter into the pan. It should be enough to form a 6 inch crepe. Cook for 2 or so minutes and then flip to cook for one more minute.

Remove it and place on a warm plate in a stack. In the end, you should be having roughly 8 crepes.

In the meantime, mix your cinnamon and sweetener in a baggie or a small bowl until well integrated.

Add half of the mixture to the softened butter as you stir until the final mixture is smooth.

Spread 1 tablespoon of the butter mixture onto the center of the crepe to serve.

Now roll up and sprinkle with one teaspoon of extra sweetener or cinnamon mixture.

Nutritional information per serving:

Calories: 434

Fat: 42g

Carbs: 2g

Protein: 12g

Salted Caramel Custard (Low Carb)

Serves 2

Ingredients

Custard:

2 eggs

1 cup water

1 1/2 teaspoon caramel extract

2 oz. cream cheese, softened

1 1/2 tablespoon granulated sugar substitute (splenda, ideal, swerve, etc.)

Caramel sauce:

2 tablespoons salted butter

1/4 teaspoon (or more, to taste) caramel extract

2 tablespoons granulated sugar substitute

Directions

For the custard, add all the five ingredients to a magic bullet or blender and blend until smooth. Grease two bowls or ramekins (6 oz.) and pour the mixture into each one.

Preheat your oven to 325 degrees F and place your ramekins in a cookie sheet and put it in the oven. Pour some hot water into this sheet until halfway up the ramekins' sides.

Bake until set, which should be about half an hour. Remove and leave to cool overnight, or chill for one hour before you serve.

For the sauce, just melt the caramel flavoring, sweetener and butter for 30 seconds in the microwave, or on a stove using a saucepan until it melts. Whisk together properly until it becomes completely blended, and then divide between the two custards and pour right before you serve.

Nutritional information per serving:

Calories: 273

Fat: 27g

Carbs: 1.5g

Protein: 9g

Delicious And Quick Lunch Soups

Tomato Soup With Cheese Croutons

Serves: 4

Ingredients

28 oz. crushed tomatoes

2 tablespoons onions, finely diced

1 clove garlic, finely chopped

1/2 cup heavy whipping cream

1 cup chicken broth

2 tablespoons fresh parsley or basil, chopped

1 cup cheddar cheese

Nonstick cooking spray

1/4 teaspoon garlic powder

Salt and pepper to taste

Directions

Spray your baking sheet using non-stick cooking spray or oil liberally. Mound the shredded cheese into tiny piles, making sure to keep not less than 1.5" between each one of them as they will spread during baking.

Sprinkle the small piles with some garlic powder and then bake for 5-6 minutes at 350 degrees F. Watch them closely. When you see the cheesing taking on a light brown color at the edges, pull them and set aside as you prepare your soup.

Get a pot and place it over medium heat. Add the chopped garlic, onions and extra-virgin olive oil. Let them cook until aromatic, for two minutes, while being careful not to let them burn.

When the onion becomes soft, add the crushed tomatoes and let simmer for roughly five minutes so that it takes on the garlic and onion flavors. Add the chicken broth bit by bit while stirring and allow to simmer for 5 more minutes.

Reduce the heat to low and add the cream while stirring. Use pepper and salt to season and then garnish with parsley leaves or basil leaves. Top with cheddar crisps, serve and enjoy!

Nutritional information per serving

Calories: 304

Fat: 27.6g

Carbs: 7.6g

Protein: 13.2g

Keto No-Noodle Chicken Soup

Serves 8

Ingredients

4 oz. butter

6 oz. sliced mushrooms

2 tablespoons dried minced onion

1 teaspoon salt

8 cups chicken broth

2 cups green cabbage sliced into strips

2 celery stalks

2 minced garlic cloves

2 teaspoons dried parsley

¼ teaspoon ground black pepper

1½ shredded rotisserie chickens

1 medium sized carrot

Directions

Start by melting the butter in a sizeable pot.

Slice the mushrooms and celery stalks into tiny bits

Add the celery, dried onion, garlic and mushrooms into the pot and cook for about three or four minutes.

Now add the parsley, carrot, broth, salt and pepper, and then simmer until the veggies become tender.

Add cabbage and cooked chicken then simmer for 8-12 more minutes until the cabbage noodles become tender.

***Nutritional information* per serving**

Calories: 509

Fat: 40g

Carbs: 4g

Protein 33g

Creamy Garlic Chicken Soup

Serves 4

Ingredients

2 tablespoons butter

4 ounces cream cheese cubed

14.5 oz. chicken broth

1/4 cup heavy cream

2 cups shredded chicken/ 1 large chicken breast

2 tablespoons Garlic Seasoning

Salt to taste

Instructions

Place a saucepan over medium heat and melt the butter.

Place the chicken in the pan and coat it with the melted butter.

As the chicken warms up, add the cream cheese cubes and the garlic seasoning and mix properly to incorporate the ingredients.

When the cream cheese melts and gets evenly distributed, just add the chicken broth and heavy cream. Bring them to a boil and then reduce the heat to low simmer for 3-4 minutes.

You can now add some salt to taste and serve.

Nutritional information per serving

Calories: 307

Fat: 25g

Carbs: 2g

Protein: 18g

Slow Cooker Low Carb Zuppa Toscana Soup

Serves 10

Ingredients

1 pound mild or hot ground Italian sausage

½ cup (1 medium) finely diced onion

36 ounces vegetable or chicken stock

3 cups chopped kale

1 teaspoon salt

½ cup heavy cream

1 tablespoon oil

3 garlic cloves, minced

1 large cauliflower head that has been diced into small florets

¼ teaspoon crushed red pepper flakes

½ teaspoon pepper

Directions

Place a skillet over medium heat and brown the ground sausage until it is ready. Remove the sausage using a slotted spoon and put it into a 6-quart slow cooker, and then discard the grease.

Add the oil to the same skillet and then sauté the onions until they turn translucent, which is about 3-4 minutes.

Put the chicken or vegetable stock, onions, kale, cauliflower florets, crushed red pepper flakes, pepper and salt to the slow cooker. Mix them properly until they are well integrated.

Let it cook on high for about 4 hours or on low for about 8 hours.

Serve hot and enjoy.

Nutritional information per serving

Calories: 246

Fat: 19g

Carbs: 7g

Protein: 14g

Keto Broccoli Cheddar Soup

Serves 4 (each serving measures 3/4 cup)

Ingredients

2 tablespoons butter

1/2 teaspoon garlic, finely minced

Salt and pepper, to taste

1 tablespoon cream cheese

1 cup cheddar cheese; shredded

1/2 teaspoon xanthan gum for thickening (optional)

1/ 8 cup white onion

2 cups of chicken broth

1 cup of chopped broccoli

1/4 cup heavy whipping cream

2 slices bacon; well cooked and crumbled (optional)

Directions

Add the butter, garlic and onion to a large pot and heat over medium heat until the onion turns soft and translucent.

Add the broccoli and broth to the pot and cook until the broccoli becomes tender. Add the pepper, salt and seasoning of your choice.

Place the cream cheese in a little bowl and microwave for about 30 seconds, or until they are soft and effortlessly stirred.

Add the heavy whipping cream while stirring, and then the cream cheese into the soup and bring it to a boil.

Turn off the heat and stir in the cheddar cheese quickly.

If using, add the xantham gum while stirring and then allow it to thicken.

Serve the dish with bacon crumbled if you desire.

Enjoy!

Nutritional information per serving

Calories: 285

Fat: 24g

Carbs: 3g

Protein: 12g

Breads, Pizzas And Other Meat-Free Baked Goods

Keto Bread

Makes 1 loaf (23 slices)

Ingredients

1½ cups almond flour

¼ teaspoon cream of tartar

¾ teaspoon baking soda

2 tablespoons coconut flour

6 egg whites

3–4 tablespoons butter, melted

3 teaspoons apple cider vinegar

Directions

Preheat your oven to 375 degrees F.

Whisk the eggs together and add the cream of tartar to the mixture. Whip the mixture using a hand mixture until you see soft peaks.

Now add the butter, almond flour, apple cider vinegar, baking soda and coconut flour to a powerful food processor and blend until it forms a desirable mixture.

Add the mixture to a bowl and fold it in the egg mixture.

Now pour the bread mixture into a properly greased 8x4 loaf pan.

Bake it for about 30 minutes.

Note that instead of using ¾ teaspoons of baking soda, you also have the option of using 3 teaspoons of baking powder and apple cider vinegar each.

Nutritional information per serving:

Calories: 65

Fat: 6g

Carbs: 2.4g

Protein: 3.1g

Low-Carb Pizza

Serves 1

Ingredients

3/4 cup warm water (if you are using xanthan gum or psyllium husks, use 1/2 cup warm water)

1 teaspoon white sugar (this one will not affect the ultimate product, as it will be consumed by the yeast)

2 tablespoons olive oil

1/2 cup Vital Wheat Gluten (64g). You can also use 1 tablespoon xanthan gum and 1/4 cup ground psyllium husks

1/2 teaspoon salt

1 1/2 teaspoons dry active yeast (quick-rise yeast is used in this recipe)

1/4 cup 14% sour cream (60g)

1 1/2 cups almond flour (168g)

1/4 cup coconut flour (30g)

1-2 teaspoons Italian spices (optional)

Directions

Add warm water to a large bowl, along with sugar and yeast. Let it sit for 5 or so minutes.

As you wait, mix all your dry ingredients in a different bowl, whisk using a fork and set aside.

Microwave your sour cream in a separate bowl for about 20-25 seconds, until it just warms a bit.

When the yeast foams (double-check to ensure it is not old), stir in the sour cream and olive oil well.

After that, add the flour as you stir until the dough starts forming.

Knead the dough using your hands for about 3 or 4 minutes.

Form a ball using the dough and put in a greased bowl before covering it using saran wrap. Put it in a warm place for 40 minutes. *You can preheat your oven to a low temperature for some time and then shut it off and place the dough there with the door open or closed, depending on the amount of heat there is.*

After 40 minutes, preheat your oven to 400 degrees F to have a thicker dough.

Get the dough out of the bowl – it should be roughly 1.5 times larger, or even more (or less if you are using xanthan gum/psyllium).

Line a baking sheet with parchment or grease it with oil. Place the dough on it and roll it out into any shape or thickness you desire (so you know, thinner seems to be working out for most people quite fine).

You can brush it using olive oil if you want, and top with anything you want.

Bake for 10-12 minutes until it turns a bit brown if you are targeting a thin crust. Otherwise, you can bake at between 350 and 400 degrees F. until it is partially cooked, and then add the topping and put it back in the oven at 450 degrees F. for the cooking to complete, if you want a thicker crust.

The one in this recipe is topped with a low carb barbecue sauce, grated parmesan cheese, mozzarella, garlic powder, oregano and basil.

Enjoy!

Remember that you can always make the dough ahead of time and refrigerate it until it is all set to bake, preferably the following day.

Nutritional information per 1/8 of the pizza:

Calories: 569

Fat: 16.5g

Carbs: 3.5g

Protein: 11g

Microwave Keto Bread - 90 Sec Flaxseed Bread

Yields 1 bread

Ingredients

1/4 cup flaxmeal

1/4 teaspoon baking soda

1 tablespoon unsweetened almond milk

1 teaspoon coconut flour

1/2 teaspoon apple cider vinegar

For the seed toppings

1/4 teaspoon sesame seeds

1/4 teaspoon pumpkin seeds

1/4 teaspoon poppy seeds

1/4 teaspoon sunflower seed

Directions

Add the flax meal, apple cider vinegar, coconut flour and unsweetened almond milk to a mixing bowl.

Using your hand, bring together the ingredients and form a ball- this should take at most one minute. At first, you may find the dough a bit sticky but still able to form into a bread ball. However, if you find it too dry, you can add some more almond milk, ½ teaspoon each time. This may take place when you use fresh grounded flaxseed that can be finer to absorb liquid slightly more.

Mix the seed on a plate and put the bread ball on the seed; press to flatten the dough, and on one side, stick the seed. Do the same on the other side. In the end, you should be having bread that is 1 cm thick, which has seeds on both sides.

Now put the bread on a plate and microwave for a minute, on high. If you want your bread to be tough or hard, you can extend the time by 20 seconds.

Remove the bread from the microwave and cool it down for a minute on the rack. Note that the bottom of the bread sitting on the plate will always be slightly moist; that is normal so don't worry when you notice it. It will quickly become dry on the rack.

Now slice your bread half and enjoy with your favorite sugar free sweetener and nut butter. You can feel free to toast the slices of bread in your toaster for more crispness. Toast on high for one minute using the bagel mode.

This bread does not store more than one hour. It is better to prepare your bread before you eat it, as the texture will change as time passes. You can just mix all the dry ingredients the day before, add the almond milk in the morning and it will be ready in 1 minute 30 seconds.

Microwave not available?

If you don't have a microwave, you can bake your bread in the oven at 360 degrees C for 8-12 minutes. Just ensure you put your bread on a baking rack well covered with parchment paper. This method will make your bread more crispier and will store better than the one prepared with a microwave. Therefore, if you want to make some bread for lunch sandwich ahead of time, you may want to go with this option.

Nutritional information per serving:

Calories: 237

Fat: 18.1g

Carbs: 13.7g

Protein: 8.3g

Vegetarian Keto Pizza Recipe

Serves 4

Ingredients

Pizza

1/2 cup almond flour (60 g)

1 tablespoon nutritional yeast (2 g)

1 egg, whisked

2 tablespoons flax meal (14 g)

1 tablespoons olive oil (15 ml)

Salt and pepper, to taste

Pizza toppings

1/4 cup keto pizza sauce (60 ml)

1 tablespoon nutritional yeast (2 g)

2 tablespoons cashew butter (30 ml)

6 basil leaves, chopped

Directions

Preheat your oven to 400 degrees F.

Mix all the first six ingredients into a dough and roll out into a flat, round pizza crust.

Now bake for about 15 minutes. After 10 minutes, flip the crust carefully.

Mix the cashew butter and pizza sauce together, and spread it over the pizza crust.

Sprinkle the top with chopped basil.

Nutritional information per serving:

Calories: 198

Fat: 16g

Carbs: 4g

Protein: 8g

Fish, Salads And Fish Salads

Avocado BLT Salad With Sweet Onion Bacon Ranch Dressing

Serves 2

Ingredients

<u>For the dressing:</u>

4 strips bacon

2 tablespoons diced onion

1 tablespoon mayonnaise

1 tablespoon water*

½ teaspoon garlic powder

¼ teaspoon pepper

1 tablespoon grease

2 teaspoons sour cream

2 tablespoons heavy cream

½ teaspoon minced fresh dill

¼ teaspoon salt

<u>For the salad</u>

4 cups chopped romaine lettuce

2 ounces cherry tomatoes

½ medium avocado, sliced

NOTE: If you prefer to have a pourable or drippy dressing, you may want to thin with 1 or 2 tablespoons of water. This particular dressing can get very thick as a result of the generous addition of the bacon grease.

Directions

Put the bacon into a skillet and fry it over medium-low heat. When both sides of the bacon become crisp, remove it from the pan to cool. Chop the bacon and set aside, until you finally become able to bring together your salad.

Now add the onion to the pan and using the rest of the bacon fat, cook on medium heat to caramelize it. Mix the onion and bacon drippings in a bowl or jar along with the dressing ingredients to make the dressing.

Mix them thoroughly. The dressing will be extremely thick due to the mayo and bacon fat. If you want to have a thinner dressing, you can thin the mixture with water.

Get a large bowl and layer your avocado, bacon, cherry tomatoes and romaine leaves salad and then drizzle the dressing and serve.

Enjoy!

Nutritional information per serving:

Calories: 338

Fat: 30.22g

Carbs: 4.86g

Protein: 8.14g

Five Minute Marinated Feta & Sun-Dried Tomato Salad

Serves 2

Ingredients

2 ounces feta, cubed

¼ teaspoon dried basil

¼ teaspoon garlic powder

2 teaspoons lemon juice

1 ounce slivered almonds

15 grams sun-dried tomatoes, diced

¼ teaspoon dried oregano

3 tablespoons olive oil

4 cups spring mix leafy greens

Salt and pepper to taste

Directions

Mix the sun dried tomatoes, herbs, cubed feta and 2/3 of the olive oil and then coat the feta in oil and herbs by tossing gently.

Let the feta marinate as you wash and prep your almonds and greens, something that should take about five minutes.

Get two small bowls or one large bowl and place your greens on top with the slivered almonds and marinated feta.

Now drizzle the rest of the olive oil and lemon juice all over the greens and then toss gently to coat.

Season with pepper and salt to taste and enjoy!

Nutritional information per serving:

Calories: 370

Fat: 33.78g

Carbs: 7.35g

Protein: 9.22g

Chicken Salad Stuffed Avocado

Serves 1

Ingredients

3 oz. chicken breast, cooked and shredded

1 stalk celery

1/3 cup sour cream

1 tablespoon red onion, diced

1 medium avocado

Directions

Start by cooking the chicken breast until well cooked, on low heat. Shred it with two forks.

Mix the chicken, celery and red onion in a bowl. Cut an avocado and pit it, and then scoop some of it into the bowl. Now add in the sour cream and then season with pepper and salt.

Toss everything properly and scoop the mix into the avocado halves.

Nutritional information per serving

Calories: 570

Fat: 45g

Carbs: 5g

Protein: 29g

Grilled Halloumi Salad

Serves 1

Ingredients

3 oz. halloumi cheese

5 grape tomatoes

5 oz. chopped walnuts

Balsamic vinegar

1 persian cucumber

1 handful baby arugula

Olive oil

Salt

Directions

Cut the cheese into slices each measuring 1/3 inches. Don't make them too thin because that would make them shrink a bit in the grill.

Grill the halloumi for 6-10 minutes on both sides. You should be able to see some grill marks along the sides.

Wash the salad and cut your veggies as a preparation for the salad; the tomatoes should be sliced in half and the cucumbers into small bits. Now chop the walnuts and mix them in a salad bowl.

Wash the arugula and add it to the bowl too.

When you notice nice, visible grill marks on both sides of the halloumi, layer it on top of your salad, sprinkle a bit of salt and dress it with balsamic vinegar and olive oil.

Serve and enjoy!

Nutritional information per serving

Calories: 560

Fat: 47g

Carbs: 7g

Protein: 21g

Keto Lemon Garlic Ghee Salmon With Leek Asparagus Ginger Saute

Serves 2

Ingredients

Lemon garlic ghee salmon

2 filets of salmon (with the skin), frozen or fresh (340 g), defrost if frozen

4 cloves garlic, minced (12 g)

Salt to taste

1 tablespoon ghee (use avocado oil for AIP)

2 teaspoons lemon juice

Lemon slices

Leek asparagus ginger sauté

10 spears of asparagus, chopped into small pieces (160 g)

2 teaspoons ginger powder (or finely diced fresh ginger if accessible)

1 tablespoon lemon juice

1 leek, chopped into small pieces (90 g)

Avocado oil or olive oil to sauté

Salt to taste

Directions

Preheat your oven to 400 degrees F.

Place the salmon filets on individual pieces of parchment paper or aluminum foils.

Divide the lemon juice, minced garlic and ghee between both filets, and place them on top of the salmon. Sprinkle with a bit of salt and then wrap up the salmon in the foil and put it in the oven.

After 10 minutes in the oven, open the foil up and bake for 10 more minutes.

As the salmon cooks, add 1 – 2 tablespoons of olive oil or avocado oil into a frying pan, add the leek and chopped asparagus and sauté on high heat. After sautéing for 10 minutes, add in the lemon juice, ginger powder and salt to taste. Sauté for another minute.

To serve, divide the sauté between 2 plates and place a filet on top of each one.

Nutritional information per serving:

Calories: 680

Fat: 51g

Carbs: 11g

Protein: 43g

Keto Baked Fish With Lemon Butter Sauce

Serves 2

Ingredients

2 (150 gram) white fish fillets

1 teaspoon salt

1 bunch broccolini

1 teaspoon garlic paste

1 tablespoon olive oil

1/2 teaspoon pepper

100 grams butter

Directions

Start by preheating your oven to 220 degrees C. Line your baking dish using baking paper and then grate the rind of the lemon finely- cut half of it into little segments. Pat dry the fish and season with pepper and salt. Using half of the lemon rind and olive oil, drizzle and put it in the oven. Bake until cooked through and just falling apart. This should take 12-14 minutes.

Put the broccolini in the microwave and steam it until it is just tender- this should take roughly 4 minutes. Drain and give it a moment to dry.

In the meantime, heat the butter in a frying pan over medium heat, until it just turns golden; this should take between 3 and 4 minutes. Now add the garlic and lemon rind and cook for one more minute. Add the steamed broccolini and lemon segments as you stir.

Serve the fish on cauliflower mash topped with lemon sauce and broccolini.

Nutritional information per serving:

Calories: 461

Fat: 47g

Carbs: 7g

Protein: 3g

Best Keto Tuna Salad

Serves 1

Ingredients

1 can tuna

2 slices bacon

1 tablespoon mayo

2 teaspoons Dijon mustard

1 large boiled egg, chopped

1 tablespoon chopped onion

1 tablespoon sour cream

1/4 teaspoon dill

Directions

Start by cooking the bacon, boiling the egg and chopping the onion.

Open the tuna, drain and put it into a little bowl.

Add the egg and chopped onion.

Add the rest of the ingredients and combine thoroughly.

Top with crumbled bacon; serve and enjoy!

Nutritional information per serving:

Calories: 298

Fat: 23g

Carbs: 1g

Protein: 21g

Paleo Sardine Stuffed Avocado

Serves 1

Ingredients

1 large avocado, seed removed (7.1 oz.)

1 tablespoon mayonnaise (0.5 oz.)

1 tablespoon fresh lemon juice

1/4 teaspoon salt

1 tin sardines, drained (3.2 oz.)

1 medium spring onion or bunch chives (0.5 oz.)

1/4 teaspoon turmeric powder/ 1 teaspoon freshly ground turmeric root

Directions

Start by halving the avocado and removing the seed. Place the drained sardines in a bowl and using a fork, break them into little pieces.

Now scoop out the center of the avocado, but leave ½ or 1 inch of its flesh. Add the finely sliced spring to the bowl of sardines along with the turmeric root or turmeric powder. Add the mayo and mix well to combine.

Add the avocado flesh you scooped and mash it into a desired consistency. Add the fresh lemon juice to the mixture and season with salt. Add the avocado mixture into each avocado half. Serve and enjoy!

Nutritional information per serving:

Calories: 633

Fat: 52.6g

Carbs: 19.5g

Protein: 27.2g

Keto Creamy Crab Salad

Serves 6

Ingredients

2 tablespoons unsalted butter

2 large cloves garlic, crushed

½ cup sour cream

2 tablespoons of fresh parsley, chopped

¾ teaspoon Old Bay Spice Mix

8 oz. lump crab meat

1 teaspoon of fresh lemon juice

½ small onion, finely diced

4 oz. cream cheese, at room temperature

4 tablespoons mayo

1 scallion, thinly sliced

1½ teaspoons fresh dill or ½ teaspoon dried dill

½ teaspoon Worcestershire sauce

2 large stalks celery, thinly sliced

Directions

Heat the butter in a little skillet over medium heat. Next, add the onion and cook, stirring occasionally until it becomes soft, but not brownish; this should take 3 minutes. Add the garlic and cook for one more minute, this time stirring frequently.

Place the onion mixture in a large bowl and add the sour cream, cream cheese, parsley, lemon juice, mayo, Worcestershire, Old Bay and scallion as you stir. Next, add the celery and crab as you stir.

Serve chilled and enjoy!

Nutritional information per serving:

Calories: 242

Fat: 21.2g

Carbs: 3.3g

Protein: 9g

Easy keto egg salad

Serves 2

Ingredients

1 avocado, medium

Splash of lemon juice

6 eggs

1/8 teaspoon dill (optional)

1/3 cup mayonnaise

1/2 tablespoon fresh chopped parsley (optional)

1 teaspoon Dijon mustard

Salt and pepper, to taste

Instructions

Put the eggs into a saucepan and cover with water. Turn on the heat and bring to a boil. Cover and leave to rest in hot water for about 10-15 minutes. You can either add more or less according to your preference.

Run the eggs under cold water for a while and then peel the shells.

Cut the eggs into tiny pieces and sprinkle with pepper and salt, and then set aside.

Mash the avocado and sprinkle with pepper and salt.

Mix the mayo, mashed avocado, mustard, any desired herbs, lemon and the eggs.

Chill, serve and enjoy!

Nutritional information per serving:

Calories: 575

Fat: 51g

Carbs: 2g

Protein: 2g

5 Ingredient Keto Chicken Salad

Serves 2

Ingredients

2 chicken breasts, boneless with the skin on (10 oz.)

1 large avocado, sliced (7.1 oz.)

4 cups of your preferred mixed greens (4.2 oz.)

4 tablespoons Paleo Ranch Dressing (you can also make your own)

Ghee or duck fat to grease

Salt and pepper, to taste

Directions

Preheat your oven to 400 degrees F. Crisp the chicken breasts up and then season the chicken breasts with pepper and salt from all sides. Grease a little skillet with duck fat or ghee. Place the chicken breasts on the hot pan, skin facing down.

Cook the chicken on high heat without moving it until it turns golden brown and crispy. This should take 5 or 6 minutes. After that, flip the chicken on the other side and cook for 30 seconds. Now move the skillet into your oven and cook it for 10- 15 minutes.

You can bake the bacon in the oven, just line a baking sheet with parchment paper and spread the slices over it. Bake for about 10 minutes, or until golden brown and crispy.

If you want, you can crisp up your bacon using a frying pan.

When the chicken cooks, move it to a cutting board and leave it to cool for about 5 minutes.

Now slice the cooked chicken and the avocado, and then assemble the salad, starting with the leafy greens followed by the avocado, crispy bacon and finally the sliced chicken.

Now top each salad with the Ranch Dressing.

NOTE: you should make sure to serve this salad immediately. Also, you can keep a bit of cooked chicken as well as the crisped up bacon in the fridge and use cold, or reheat if preferred.

Nutritional information per serving:

Calories: 581

Fat: 43.8g

Carbs: 10.5g

Protein: 38.7g

Conclusion

We have come to the end of the book. Thank you for reading and congratulations for reading until the end.

The book has been your way to ensure your lunch and dinner meals are healthy and delightful all at the same time. Most of these recipes are simple to prepare and take a few minutes to execute and all this work is devoted to making sure you don't have an excuse to not live longer, lose weight and enjoy all the other benefits good keto friendly food can offer.

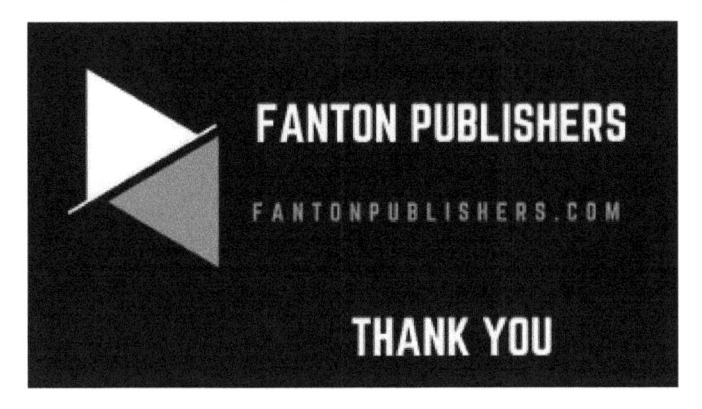

Do You Like My Book & Approach To Publishing?

If you like my writing and style and would love the ease of learning literally everything you can get your hands on from Fantonpublishers.com, I'd really need you to do me either of the following favors.

1: First, I'd Love It If You Leave a Review of This Book on Amazon.

2: Check Out My Other Keto Diet Books

KETOGENIC DIET: Keto Diet Made Easy: Beginners Guide on How to Burn Fat Fast With the Keto Diet (Including 100+ Recipes That You Can Prepare Within 20 Minutes)- New Edition

KETOGENIC DIET: Ketogenic Diet Recipes That You Can Prepare Using 7 Ingredients and Less in Less Than 30 Minutes

Ketogenic Diet: With A Sustainable Twist: Lose Weight Rapidly With Ketogenic Diet Recipes You Can Make Within 25 Minutes

Ketogenic Diet: Keto Diet Breakfast Recipes

Fat Bombs: Keto Fat Bombs: 50+ Savory and Sweet Ketogenic Diet Fat Bombs That You MUST Prepare Before Any Other!

Snacks: Keto Diet Snacks: 50+ Savory and Sweet Ketogenic Diet Snacks That You MUST Prepare Before Any Other!

Desserts: Keto Diet Desserts: 50+ Savory and Sweet Ketogenic Diet Desserts That You MUST Prepare Before Any Other!

Ketogenic Diet: Ketogenic Diet Lunch and Dinner Recipes

Ketogenic Diet: Keto Diet Cookbook For Vegetarians

Ketogenic Diet: Ketogenic Slow Cooker Cookbook: Keto Slow Cooker Recipes That You Can Prepare Using 7 Ingredients Or Less

Note: This list may not represent all my Keto diet books. You can check the full list by visiting my Author Central: amazon.com/author/fantonpublishers or my website http://www.fantonpublishers.com

Get updates when we publish any book on the Ketogenic diet: http://bit.ly/2fantonpubketo

Closely related to the keto diet is intermittent fasting. I also publish books on Intermittent Fasting.

One of the books is shown below:

Intermittent Fasting: A Complete Beginners Guide to Intermittent Fasting For Weight Loss, Increased Energy, and A Healthy Life

Get updates when we publish any book on intermittent fasting: http://bit.ly/2fantonbooksIF

To get a list of all my other books, please fantonwriters.com, my author central or let me send you the list by requesting them below: http://bit.ly/2fantonpubnewbooks

3: Let's Get In Touch

Antony

Website: http://www.fantonpublishers.com/

Email: Support@fantonpublishers.com

Twitter: https://twitter.com/FantonPublisher

Facebook Page: https://www.facebook.com/Fantonpublisher/

My Ketogenic Diet Books Page: https://www.facebook.com/pg/Fast-Keto-Meals-336338180266944

Private Facebook Group For Readers: https://www.facebook.com/groups/FantonPublishers/

Pinterest: https://www.pinterest.com/fantonpublisher/

4: Grab Some Freebies On Your Way Out; Giving Is Receiving, Right?

I gave you 2 freebies at the start of the book, one on general life transformation and one about the Ketogenic diet. Grab them here if you didn't grab them earlier.

Ketogenic Diet Freebie: http://bit.ly/2fantonpubketo

5 Pillar Life Transformation Checklist: http://bit.ly/2fantonfreebie

5: Suggest Topics That You'd Love Me To Cover To Increase Your Knowledge Bank.

I am looking forward to seeing your suggestions and insights; you could even suggest improvements to this book. Simply send me a message on Support@fantonpublishers.com.

PSS: Let Me Also Help You Save Some Money!

If you are a heavy reader, have you considered subscribing to Kindle Unlimited? You can read this and millions of other books for just $9.99 a month)! You can check it out by searching for Kindle Unlimited on Amazon!

Milton Keynes UK
Ingram Content Group UK Ltd.
UKHW010637260923
429409UK00001B/165